How to lose weight, gain energy and detoxify your body in 10 days

By Janie L. Hobbs

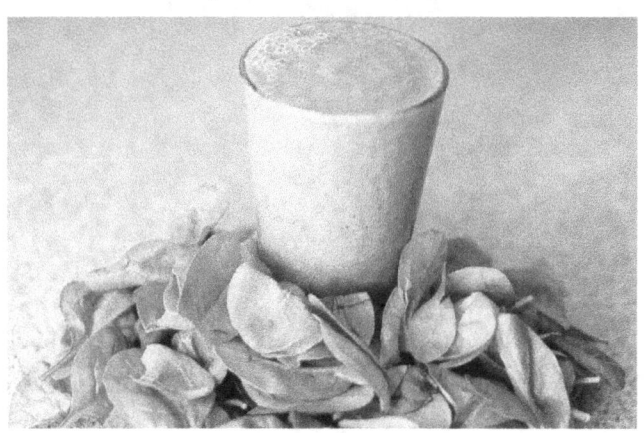

ഋ ഋ ഋ

"I lost 18 lbs. on this green smoothie regiment in 10 days"
Janie

Nutrition is my mission!

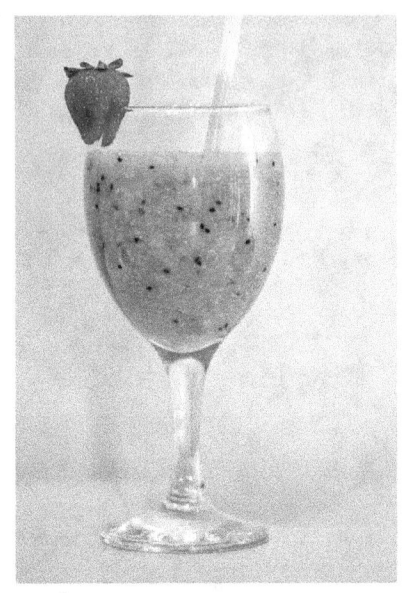

THE POWER OF DETOXING AND DRINKING GREEN VEGETABLES AND FRUIT SMOOTHIES TO CLEANSE YOUR BODY

FOREWORD

For me this little book is a dream come true. So many of my friends and associates have asked me over the years for information regarding herbs, smoothies, and home remedies for various ailments that they have been faced with. I have finally decided after a request from my loving and understanding husband along with the desire in my heart, to put this information in booklet form and leave it as a legacy so others may benefit from it in years to come   So, this book is dedicated first to God, my husband Allen, my wonderful children, and my adorable grandchildren.

Happy cleansing and weight loss and enjoy the new you!

Janie Hobbs

Janie Hobbs

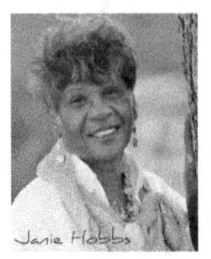

Janie Hobbs

JANIE HOBBS BIO

Janie Hobbs is a Nutrition Specialist who believes in herbal remedies, vegetable smoothies and natural treatments along with Lifestyle Health Coaching for cleansing, weight loss and healing of the human body. She is a minister and spiritual life coach, retired licensed cosmetologist, very knowledgeable in the area of health and physical fitness and Al-anon serenity for co-dependents.

She holds a bachelor's degree in theology and a certificate in food nutrition and health.

Janie was born in Wetumpka, Alabama and shortly thereafter her family moved to Los Angeles, California where she grew up.

Janie is a well-rounded individual who has helped many people lose weight, cleanse their bodies, and feel more energized. She has spoken at several events and has conducted many seminars on health and nutrition. She lives with passion dedication and grace, is the wife of Allen J. Hobbs Jr., the mother of 9 children and a very proud grandmother.

Acknowledgements

My first appreciation is to my loving husband who has unfailingly supported and encouraged me through the writing of this book. My beautiful daughter Angie and my wonderful son in-law Senai, my son Allen (Tom) who were there for me as I shared ideas for this book with them. And my 2 granddaughters, Aaliyah and Kendall who continues to be my best cheerleaders.

"Go Mema go"

As you know it is very difficult for most people to lose weight, they approach it with the best intentions but their schedules and their lifestyle makes it hard for them to lose the weight and get rid of those toxins that make it so hard for us to avoid many diseases.

Here is a way to kick start your weight loss and start the detoxifying process!

The Green and fruit Smoothie Cleanse is a 3, 5 or 10-Day detox cleanse that consists of green leafy veggies, fruits and water, (no juices) These smoothies pack a lot of nourishment for your body and they are very, very healthy, purifying your body, rebuilding itself from the inside out.

Not a diet

This fruit and vegetable detox cleanse is not a diet, but it provides a natural plan of nourishing, purifying and maintaining healthy lifestyle. Your major organ systems will be supported with vitamins, minerals and nutrients that is in natural raw foods. Your body will thank you for drinking them. You will lose some weight, your energy levels will increase, your cravings will greatly reduce, your mind will be clear, your digestion and overall health will be enhanced. This experience will change your life if you stick with it. Aside from losing weight it will improve diabetes, cholesterol, high blood pressure, and thyroid, curve your appetite, increase your energy and will improve on many other diseases.

The Reason for detoxing and cleansing the body and drinking herbal teas

Detox and herbal teas are known to flush toxic fats from your body, while purifying it and this is all naturally. Not only does it purify the body, it also revitalizes the major organs, and curbs the appetite. That is great news for slimming because these toxins are linked to increased fat storage and metabolic slowdowns. To prevent acidic waste from damaging the thyroid and other organs, it is very important to drink detox and herbal teas to neutralize the acidic waste and improve the glands ability to speed up the metabolism.

Great improvement in health is the results your body and mind will receive from this powerful natural way of eating nutritional fruits, green vegetables and drinking these detox smoothie cleanse while sipping away at the herbal teas.

These fruits and vegetables are raw, organic and loaded with nutrient.

Because detoxing plays a major part in expelling, metabolizing and minimizing weight, you will, after the 10-day cleanse, be excited about how wonderful your body looks and how good you feel

Toxins can develop into many conditions

I have listed below the many conditions that can develop from toxins in your body:

- ✓ Reduce mental clarity
- ✓ Joint discomfort
- ✓ Skin problems
- ✓ Fibromyalgia
- ✓ Stuffy head
- ✓ Weight gain
- ✓ Difficulty sleeping
- ✓ Food craving
- ✓ Fatigue
- ✓ Headaches
- ✓ High blood pressure
- ✓ Depression
- ✓ Constipation

- ✓ Infections
- ✓ Allergies
- ✓ Gastrointestinal problems
- ✓ Thyroid problems
- ✓ Digestion problems
- ✓ Diabetes

When the body is full of toxins, it does not have the energy to burn calories therefore the above problems occur.

Before you start your detox cleanse start a daily chart

A. Weigh yourself
B. Take pictures (optional)
C. Measure yourself:
   Hips/waist/bust/chest/thighs/arms
D. Weigh yourself each day – (your weight maybe up and down as you do your cleanse, it is ok, don't panic. Remember the best news is that you are getting healthy.

Three – five – ten – day fruit, green vegetable detox herbal cleanse

This 3/5/10- day fruit, green vegetable detox herbal cleanse is an amazing nutritional healing and healthy experience.

Drink one 6oz cup of detox tea on an empty stomach. Do this daily. Prepare herb tea, smoothies or other food for the day.

"Nutrition is my mission"

Now! Let's get started on making nutrition your mission for the next 3/5/or 10 days!!

How to prepare ten day fruit and vegetable smoothies

Some of you might be working or have other reasons to be away from home during the day. If this is the case, you will need to prepare smoothies, teas, water and snacks for the day, and keep refrigerated.

11

Prepare enough for 3 smoothies, 3 herbal teas, and 3 detox teas every day, make sure to drink 6-8 glasses of water to help flush out toxins. This is necessary for cleansing the colon.

You may snack on apples, celery, carrots, cucumbers, and raw unsalted nuts and seeds only a handful.

How to do a 3-5 day light cleanse

Drink two 6oz cups of detox tea a day, three 6oz cups herb tea a day, two fruit and vegetable smoothies a day. If you get hungry, you may have a small snack, green salad with lunch. Drink 6 to 8 glasses of water a day.

Herbal Teas

Here are some detox teas you may purchase for detox the body and cleansing the colon. Listed below are some suggested brands:

Yogi Brand – is organic detox and is a gentle way to help the body cleanse itself by aiding the liver and the kidneys. Yogi detox have a variety of flavors: plain, berry, peach, roasted dandelion spice.

Gaia Brand -   Herbal Teas is an excellent herbal tea, with each brewed cup delivering a delicious taste experience as well as fast-acting support. Gaia brand of teas are organic and good for everyday cleanse.

Alvita Brand – These teas are organic or caffeine free, with a variety of flavors such as: ginger root, green tea, peppermint, chamomile, dandelion root, red clover, alfalfa leaf, valerian root, paud,arco, rosemary leaf, fennel, hawthorn berries, mullein leaf, black tea, Gardena tea.

When sweetening your tea you may use one or two teaspoons of 100% pure raw and unfiltered honey or one or two packets of Stevia in the raw 100% natural zero calorie sugar.

Do not eat the items below on your three, five, or ten-day cleanse

Donuts, Ice cream, cake, cheese, meat, processed food, fried foods, white bread, pasta, refined sugar, milk, coffee, beer, liquor, sodas, diet sodas, chips, candy.

If you get hungry and need food you may eat the following:

Fish: When you purchase fish of any kind, make sure it is not farm raised, it should always be "wild caught"

Chicken Breast should be skinless and boneless, baked or grilled.

Green salad, no salt please

Steamed or raw vegetables, cabbage, green beans, spinach, collard greens, kale, turnip greens, chards, eggplant, asparagus, Brussel sprouts, okra, cauliflower, broccoli, mushrooms, kelp,

No Salt Please!!!

Here are some seasonings that should be used when seasoning your meals:

- ✓ Mrs. Dash salt-free onion and herb
- ✓ Mrs. Dash salt free garlic and herb
- ✓ Rosemary, Basil, Fennel seed, Parsley, Oregano, Thyme, Turmeric, Garlic Pepper, Cayenne Pepper, Cumin Seed. Coriander and Bay leaves.

A message for the Diabetic

People with diabetes cannot have a lot of certain fruits. When making smoothies you can add less fruit to the smoothie to make sure not to raise your sugar level. The key is to keep an eye on portion sizes and stay away from fruits canned in syrups or other types of added sugar. When adding sugar to the smoothie, be sure to use one tablespoon 100% pure raw & unfiltered honey or two packets of Stevia sweetener.

Blending: If you have a small blender you may have to make the smoothie in two batches, have a pitcher on hand since you are going to be making enough for the whole day, make sure you add a few ice cubes to the smoothie in the blender for thickness.

And now let's begin!

Day 1: Spinach/Strawberries

- ❖ 1 cup of spring mix
- ❖ 2 cups of spinach
- ❖ 1 cup of bananas fresh or frozen
- ❖ 2 cups of strawberries
- ❖ 1 cup blueberries fresh or frozen
- ❖ 1 cup of apples peeled and cut up
- ❖ 1 stevia packet if necessary
- ❖ 2 cups of water
- ❖ 1 small avocado, peeled, seeded and cut up
- ❖ 2 tablespoons organic ground chia seeds
- ❖ 2 tablespoons organic raw-unfiltered apple cider vinegar

Place all items and 2 cups of water in blender and blend until creamy

Day 2- Apple/Pineapple/Grape

- ❖ 2 cups of spring mix greens
- ❖ 2 cups of water
- ❖ 1 cup spinach
- ❖ 1 banana pealed
- ❖ 2 cups of strawberries
- ❖ 1 ½ cups of frozen pineapple
- ❖ 1 cup of apples
- ❖ 1 cup of grapes
- ❖ 2 tablespoons organic ground chia seeds
- ❖ 1 teaspoon organic ground cinnamon

Place leafy greens and water in blender and blend for 30 seconds. Add all Ingredients and blend.

Day 3- Strawberry/Peach/Lemon

- ❖ 2 cups of spinach
- ❖ 1 cup of Kale
- ❖ 2 cups of water
- ❖ 2 sprigs of fresh cilantro (if organic ground, 1 tablespoon)

17

- ❖ 2 cups of strawberries(frozen)
- ❖ 2 cups of peaches (frozen)
- ❖ 1 cup of bananas (frozen or fresh)
- ❖ 2 tablespoons of organic ground chia seeds
- ❖ 2 tablespoon 100% lemon juice
- ❖ 1 tablespoon 100% pure raw unfiltered honey
- ❖ 1 teaspoon organic ground turmeric

Place water and green vegetables in blender and blend for 30 seconds. Add all of the other ingredients and blend.

Day 4- Kale/Spinach/Fruit mix

- ❖ 2 cups of spinach
- ❖ 3 cups of kale
- ❖ 2 cups of water
- ❖ 3 ½ cups of frozen mixed fruit
- ❖ 1 banana (frozen or fresh)
- ❖ 1 tablespoon 100% pure raw and unfiltered honey
- ❖ 2 tablespoons organic ground chia seeds
- ❖ 2 sprigs of fresh parsley or organic ground

- ❖ ¼ teaspoon organic cayenne pepper
- ❖ 2 tablespoons 100% lemon juice

Place water and green vegetables in blender and blend for 30 seconds. Add all of the other ingredients and blend.

Day 5 – Green vegetable Mango Delight

- ❖ 2 cups of kale
- ❖ 2 cups of spinach
- ❖ 2 cups of water
- ❖ 1 apple
- ❖ 1 ½ cups of mangos (frozen)
- ❖ 1 ½ cups of strawberries (frozen)
- ❖ 1 banana
- ❖ 1 cup blueberries (frozen)
- ❖ 2 tablespoons organic ground chia seeds
- ❖ 2 tablespoons organic raw unfiltered apple cider vinegar
- ❖ 2 tablespoons organic fresh squeezed lemon juice

Place water and green vegetables in blender and blend for 30 seconds. Add all other ingredients and blend.

Day-6 Cinnamon/Berry/Supercharge

- ❖ 2 cups fresh spinach
- ❖ 1 cup of Kale
- ❖ 2 cups of water
- ❖ 3 ½ cups mixed berries (frozen)
- ❖ 2 bananas
- ❖ 1cup of apples
- ❖ 1 cup of grapes
- ❖ 2 tablespoons organic ground flax seeds
- ❖ 2 teaspoons organic ground cinnamon
- ❖ 1 tablespoon nutiva hemp protein organic superfood (your choice)
- ❖ 2 teaspoons organic squeezed lemon juice

Place water and green vegetables in blender and blend for 30 seconds add all other ingredients and blend

Day 7- Blueberry/Apple blend

- ½ cup of kale
- ½ cup of spring mix
- 2 cups of water
- 1 cup of spinach
- 3 cups of blueberries (frozen)
- 1 cup of peaches frozen
- 1 cup of strawberries
- 2 cups of apples
- 1 banana
- 2 sprigs of parsley(or one tablespoon dried)
- 2 tablespoon organic ground flaxseed
- 1tablespoon Nutiva hemp protein organic superfood (your choice)
- 1 teaspoon organic ground turmeric

Place water and green vegetables in blender and blend for 30 seconds add all other ingredients and blend

Day 8- Spinach Latte

- ❖ 3 cups of spinach
- ❖ 1 cup of bananas
- ❖ 2 cups of water
- ❖ 1 cup of pineapples (frozen)
- ❖ 1 cup of peaches
- ❖ 2 cups of strawberries (frozen)
- ❖ ½ teaspoon organic ground turmeric
- ❖ 1 ½ tablespoons organic ground flaxseed
- ❖ 1 tablespoon 100% pure raw unfiltered honey
- ❖ ½ teaspoon organic ground cinnamon

Place water and greens in blender and blend for 30 seconds. Add all of the other ingredients and blend

Day 9- Spring mix Java

- ❖ 2 cups of spring mix
- ❖ 1 cup of avocado
- ❖ 2 cups of water
- ❖ 2 cups of bananas
- ❖ 1 ¼ cups of blueberries (frozen)

22

- ❖ 2 cups strawberries (frozen)
- ❖ 1 ½ cups pineapples (frozen)
- ❖ 1 tablespoons organic ground flaxseed
- ❖ 1 tablespoon organic fresh squeezed lemon juice
- ❖ ½ teaspoon organic cayenne pepper
- ❖ ½ teaspoon organic ground cinnamon
- ❖ ½ teaspoon organic raw-unfiltered apple cider vinegar
- ❖ ½ teaspoon 100% raw unfiltered honey
- ❖ ½ teaspoon organic ground turmeric

Place water and green vegetables in blender and blend for 30 seconds, add all of the other ingredients and blend

Day 10 Pineapple Strawberry Mocha

- ❖ 1 ½ cups of spinach
- ❖ 1 cup of kale
- ❖ 2 cups of water
- ❖ 2 cups of strawberries
- ❖ 1 cup of bananas

- ❖ 1 apple
- ❖ 1 ½ cups of pineapples
- ❖ 1 tablespoon organic ground flaxseed
- ❖ 1 tablespoon organic ground flaxseed
- ❖ ½ teaspoon organic ground cinnamon
- ❖ 1 teaspoon organic raw unfiltered apple cider vinegar
- ❖ 1 teaspoon 100% pure raw unfiltered honey
- ❖ ¼ teaspoon organic ground turmeric

Place water and green vegetables in blender and blend for 30 seconds. Add all of the other ingredients and blend

Continue Healthy Eating After the Cleanse

Great! Wonderful! You made it! Now it's time to continue healthy nutritional eating. You can keep the body cleansed daily, weekly, monthly if you continue to eat and drink in the correct way.

Do some type of exercise daily or at least three times a week
Start your exercise slow if you haven't exercise for a while. Eating and drinking healthy will keep those unwanted pounds off.

Here is how you keep those unwanted pounds off by watching the following items you eat

- Sugar
- Carbohydrates
- Sodium
- Fats

Note: You cannot eat pork bacon, pork sausage, grits or white rice on a regular menu.

The reason for a three – five – ten- day fruit or vegetable cleanse is the amazing results your body and mind receives from the awesome natural way of eating and drinking raw. They are loaded with nutrients, they are organic and uncooked.

Here are a few tips for the first 2 days of eating after the cleanse, remember your stomach have not had food for ten days. In order to not get stomach pain, eat very light. Broiled or baked chicken or fish, green salad, drink one smoothie per day, two herbal teas and remember to drink plenty of water.

Fruits

Strawberries, grapes, apples, pears, kiwi, blueberries, bananas, cherries and pineapples, peaches, plums, blackberries, watermelon, cantaloupe, pumpkin, honeydew melon, mangos, papayas, nectarines, avocado are also good.

Vegetables

Spinach, broccoli, green cabbage, kale, red cabbage, collard greens, turnip greens, mustard greens, eggplant, beets, green beans, green peas, mixed vegetables, cucumbers, asparagus, lettuce, mixed spring greens, artichokes, Brussel sprouts, radishes, kelp, okra, mushrooms, cauliflower, onion, celery, peppers, sweet potatoes, corn, white potatoes, beans and legumes (organic better soaked), white beans, lima beans, red beans, kidney beans, split peas, black beans, navy beans, garbanzo beans, lentils, black eyed peas, butter beans.

Meats

Fish – baked, grilled or broiled

Chicken Breast (skinless, boneless) – grilled, baked or broiled

Salmon (wild) – Baked or grilled

Ground lean chicken, ground lean turkey (97% or 98%) Lean steak, lean turkey sausage, lean turkey bacon.

Seasoning

All of the seasonings listed below should be organic:

Garlic powder, Onion powder, garlic pepper, oregano, ground turmeric, ground cinnamon, cayenne pepper, Mrs. Dash, Fennel seeds, cumin seeds, parsley, crush mint, rosemary, Italian seasonings, marjoram, lemon pepper, dill weed, curry powder. 100% coconut oil virgin & unrefined. 100% extra virgin olive oil first cold pressing.

Coconut milk Dairy free, Gluten free, soy free, non GMO

Sugar – Stevia in the raw 100% natural zero calorie sweetener.

Butter – Earth Balance

You can lose between 3 and 18 lbs. with these vegetable smoothies

The American Cancer Society recommends that we eat 5-9 servings of fruits and vegetables each day to prevent cancer and other diseases. The smoothies in this book are a quick and convenient way to get your vegetables and dark, leafy greens without tasting them. The fruit masks the flavor so even though all you taste is banana, mango, and pineapple or strawberry, you are eating a healthy dose of spinach, carrots, kale and any other vegetable that you put in.

"Nutrition is my Mission"

The smoothies in this book is the BEST ways to get amazing nutrition, detox your body and have a steady energy boost at any time of the day.

Try it! You'll like it!!!

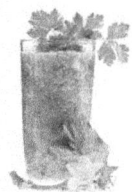

For further information contact me at jhealthandnutrition@gmail.com or visit my website at jhealthandnutrition.com

The biggest thing we're missing in our weight loss and detox regiment on a daily basis is a plan

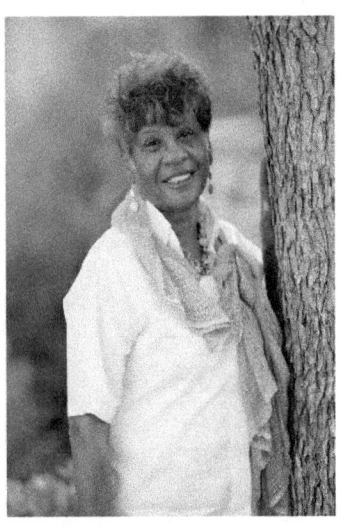

A plan that isn't complicated

A plan that can be followed even when our schedule gets busy

A plan that produces measurable results fast enough that we won't get discouraged with the process.

This **weight loss** green smoothie **book has the plan** for you

Janie Hobbs is a Nutrition Specialist who believes in herbal remedies, vegetable smoothies and natural treatments along with Lifestyle Health Coaching for cleansing, weight loss and healing of the human body. She is a minister and spiritual life coach, retired licensed cosmetologist, very knowledgeable in the area of health and physical fitness and Al-anon serenity for co-dependents. She holds a bachelor's degree in theology and a certificate in food nutrition and health. Janie was born in Wetumpka, Alabama and shortly thereafter her family moved to Los Angeles, California where she grew up.